Sugar Detox That Rocks

Proven Techniques to Defeat Your Sugar Addiction, Feel Better and Lose Weight

I0430024

Sugar Detox That Rocks
Proven Techniques to Defeat Your Sugar Addiction, Feel Better and Lose Weight

By Hanna Davis

Copyright © 2014 Softpress Publishing

All rights reserved.

Disclaimer:

Table of Contents

Introduction

Congratulations on deciding to make changes in your life toward better health!

At some point in our lives I think we all become a slave to sugar. It's just so darned good and our bodies seem to crave it more now than ever before in history. Have you ever stopped to ask yourself why this is? Are we addicted to sugar? Is it possible to *quit* sugar altogether? Well, there are no easy answers to those questions, but we are going to discuss those topics as well as others in the following chapters as I teach you how to detox your body from sugars deadly grip.

I've included a short quiz of sorts in Chapter one to help you determine if you currently have a problem with sugar in your diet. I'd recommend answering the questions honestly as you begin to read this book, then re-take the quiz after your successful detox and compare the answers. I bet you'll be surprised.

Remember, anything worth doing is worth doing well so I won't *sugar-coat* the process (that just wouldn't be right). This won't be an easy journey. However, I have confidence in you and know you will succeed. So let's jump right in and get started.

As a way of saying Thank You for buying my book I have put together a **FREE GIFT** just for you!

"8 Snack and Dessert Options for Your Sugar Detox"

This gift is the perfect complement to this book so just head over to this web address to get access

http://www.softpresspublishing.com/sugardetox/

Chapter 1 - Is Sugar Addictive?

If you are hoping to cut out refined sugar from your diet in order to be a healthier you, you have probably realized it is extremely difficult. About midday you get this strong craving for soda or a candy bar. You need something sweet. Your body will not be satisfied by a quick drink of ice water or a rice cake. It craves sugar. In fact, the craving is so strong many liken it to a drug craving or a nicotine craving.

So, is sugar addictive? This is a subject of great debate among experts. Researchers and scientists are divided on whether or not sugar is truly addictive or if the strong desire is something that could be controlled if a person tried hard enough.

Most research says it isn't addicting per se, but it is certainly something a person feels addicted to. In fact, it is subjective for each person. Scientists cannot unequivocally deny sugar has some addictive qualities, but there are plenty of experts who say it is an addiction that is all in our heads. On the flip side of the argument, a new study supports the idea that sugar is truly addictive, just like any illicit drug.[1]

According to the dictionary, addiction is defined as:

- A strong and harmful need to regularly have something (such as a drug) or do something (such as gamble).

- An unusually great interest in something or a need to do or have something.

Doesn't that sound like the way you feel about your Pepsi or your afternoon candy bar? How many times have you driven all the way to the store, maybe in your sweats and flip flops, just so you could get a soda to satisfy your sugar craving?

---

[1]http://ajcn.nutrition.org/content/early/2013/06/26/ajcn.113.064113.abstract

The bottom line is this: sugar has addictive qualities that can make it difficult to cut from our diet. Strong cravings can make us do some pretty strange things in order to get our hands on the substance. Check out the next section to see if you are battling a sugar addiction.

Signs you're addicted

Ask yourself these questions and be honest.

1 - Do you get a craving for something sweet about the same time every day? Maybe around 2 in the afternoon or just before bed?

2 - When there is a spread of food at parties or buffets, do you tend to go for the sweet foods?

3 - Do you get a headache or feel out of sorts when you try and cut out your afternoon sugar fix?

4 - Do you eat a candy bar or other foods high in sugar just because you want the sweetness and not because you are truly hungry?

5 - You need more sugar to satisfy your craving. Maybe you would eat half a donut during the day to get your sugar fix, but now you need a whole donut plus a can of soda.

6 - You overeat and end up feeling sluggish. You know you are eating too much but can't seem to stop yourself.

7 - Your sugary eating habits have led to significant weight gain and your physical and social health is suffering because of it.

8 - Do you feel guilty about the sugar you consume?

9 - Is the level of fun you have at a certain event measured by the sugary foods available?

10 - When you are feeling a little sad or down, do you crave certain foods like pizza, ice cream or chocolate?

If you answered yes to any of these questions, you are likely battling some kind of addiction to sugar or at the very least, a very strong desire to have sugar in your diet. If you are reading this, you likely feel as if you are hovering around the sugar addiction problem. Even if you don't have an actual addiction (depending on what side of **that** fence you are on) you may still be battling cravings that tend to rule your day.

Why we are addicted to sugar

Now that you have determined you certainly have a strong inkling towards sugar addiction, you need to know why. Why are you addicted to sugar? Were you born that way or is it something you did a few years back that drew you to sugar?

To answer the first question, yes. Yes, you were born with the desire for sugar. It is part of survival and our bodies are programmed to survive from the very moment we are born. Infants prefer sweeter foods and drinks over bland drinks and foods from the very hour they are born. The issue is, like with any substance, we need more and more to satisfy that craving or achieve that happy, satisfied feeling we get when that first burst of sugar hits our taste buds.

From early on, good times are associated with sugary foods. Birthday cakes, Thanksgiving feasts, Christmas dinner and other special occasions are all celebrated with food. Foods that are typically high in sugar. Those buttery rolls that are served with Thanksgiving are not candy, but they are high in sugar. Sugar is in nearly everything we eat these days. Our tolerance levels are extremely high, because of the amount of sugar we eat on a regular basis.

When we strive to reach that little bit of euphoria that a nice sugary drink or treat will give us, we have to drink a lot or eat more of it. Have you noticed the size of soft drinks lately? 20 or 30 years ago, a 20-ounce soda was enough to satisfy the need for sugar. Nowadays, you see these gallon jugs of soda with a straw sticking out of them. Instead of a single cookie, cookies are sold in 3s. We have evolved and our need for more sugar has increased exponentially. That need has made us a society of unhealthy individuals battling obesity and diabetes brought on by too much sugar.

Why do we crave sugar?

So what is it that makes us do crazy things, like beat up a vending machine that refuses to relinquish that candy bar we just paid for? It all has to do with serotonin and dopamine. These are two neurotransmitters in the brain that affect your mood. When you do things that make you feel good, your body gets a healthy dose of dopamine and your mood is elevated.

When you are feeling particularly down, your serotonin levels drop. This sends out a red alert to your body that you need something that will make you feel good and happy. That something is usually sugar. When you skip breakfast and your tummy is rumbling, you will get a craving for sugar. That is your body telling you your serotonin levels have dropped and it wants replenishment.

Have you ever noticed after a particularly sleepless night you tend to crave sugar a bit more? It isn't only for the five minute energy boost you get. It is because your body is running low on fuel and is telling you it needs something quick. Sugar and carbohydrate-laden foods, like chips and candy bars, provide that quick lift. Your brain sends out a signal that gives you that craving.

The following are three main reasons you crave sugar:

- Dehydration
- Tiredness
- Sedentary lifestyles

By making a conscience effort to get enough sleep, exercise regularly and drink plenty of water, you can help eliminate some of your sugar cravings. We will discuss this further later in the book.

Chapter 2 - Difference Between Good and Bad Sugars

It is important to understand that not all sugars are bad. Your body needs some sugar in order to function at its best. There is sugar in natural foods, like milk and fruit and then there is the sugar that we add to our food.

Bad sugar is the term used to refer to refined sugar. Sodas, cookies, breads and candy are loaded with refined sugar. This is the sugar that causes health problems and is the type of sugar you should aim to cut out or dramatically reduce the intake in your regular diet.

Sugar is sugar, but it is the way our bodies handle the sugar that makes some sugars good and other sugars bad. Sugar is made up of fructose and glucose. Both are necessary for our bodies. Fructose processes fairly easily and quickly by the liver without provoking a negative response. Glucose, on the other hand, needs insulin, which is released by the pancreas, to be broken down by the body. As you probably know, excess insulin or too little insulin can create serious problems, like diabetes.

The reason naturally occurring sugar that is found in fruits and even some vegetables is safe and better for you to eat is the fact it is bundled with plenty of good things your body needs. Fiber, along with various vitamins and minerals, helps your body digest the sugar better without the rise in insulin. You don't get that sugar high when you eat a bowl full of strawberries, but you can still satisfy your sugar craving without overworking your pancreas and causing a dangerous increase in your blood sugar.

Naturally occurring sugars that are wrapped up in fiber and vitamins are non-fattening as well, which makes them good for you. You can eat a bowl of fruit without worrying about your teeth hurting and gaining five pounds versus eating a bowl full of candy.

Artificial Sweeteners

Artificial sweeteners are often used in place of refined sugar in various products on the market. You may buy artificial sweeteners to add to your coffee and tea. Are you really helping your body by using the artificial sugars available?

This is another one of those topics where people are all for artificial sweeteners, while others prefer to skip anything that is manufactured in a lab. It is personal preference. As of now, there are no studies that prove things like Splenda or Sweet 'n' Low are dangerous or cause cancer despite the rumors. However, there are definitely some side effects associated with using artificial sweeteners. Some people get terrible stomach pain and headaches when they use artificial sweeteners.

There are plenty of different sweeteners on the market so it can be a little tough to choose which one you like best. The lists below include most of the sweeteners currently on the market and what they are made from.[2]

Artificial Sweeteners
Acesulfame potassium (Sunett, Sweet One)
Aspartame (Equal, NutraSweet)
Neotame
Saccharin (SugarTwin, Sweet'N Low)
Sucralose (Splenda)

Sugar Alcohols
Erythritol
Hydrogenated starch hydrolysate
Isomalt

---

[2]   http://www.mayoclinic.org/healthy-living/nutrition-and-healthy-eating/in-depth/artificial-sweeteners/art-20046936

Lactitol
Maltitol
Mannitol
Sorbitol
Xylitol

Novel Sweeteners
Stevia extracts (Pure Via, Truvia)
Tagatose (Naturlose)
Trehalose

Natural sweeteners
Agave nectar
Date sugar
Fruit juice concentrate
Honey
Maple syrup
Molasses

If you are not comfortable using artificial sweeteners, there are several more natural options. Honey is a favorite for teas, cookies and even pancakes. Raw honey is very sweet and is actually good for you. Agave nectar is gaining in popularity and can now be found in most grocery stores.

It is important to point out all sugar substitutes, whether they be natural or artificial, are much sweeter than refined sugar. You need a lot less to sweeten your cup of coffee.

Some experts are convinced artificial sweeteners are the way to go in the fight against obesity. They contain a fraction of the calories of refined sugar. Another benefit of the artificial varieties is they do not cause the insulin spikes. They are processed quicker by the body. Diabetics who still want to enjoy a little sweet treat can opt for one made with an artificial sweetener. However, it is crucial a person who has diabetes talks with their doctor about which sweetener is best for their situation. As with everything in life, there are some mild side effects or warnings associated with artificial sweeteners so read labels carefully.

Chapter 3 - Step by Step Detox Plan

You have made the decision to eliminate the refined sugar in your diet. You will need a detox plan that will help you through each step and outline what you can expect. There is no one size fits all. You may get through the detox without a single craving or you may be one of the few who experience strong cravings throughout the day. No matter where you fall on the detox scale, know this—**You Can Do It! And you will feel better for doing so!**

Because there is no time like the present, you can start your sugar detox right now, this very minute. If you have a soda, pour it out. Your best bet is to go cold turkey. You are in full detox mode and refined sugars and refined carbs are no longer on your list of foods to eat. It starts now. Detoxing requires you to completely eliminate all sugars from your diet for a set period. Typically, 21 days is the goal. More on this timetable later in the chapter.

How to get through Sugar Withdrawal

It is a mental battle as you tell your body you are no longer giving into those cravings for candy or soda. Set a goal. Tell yourself you will not consume refined sugar for 7 days, 72 hours or whatever you decide. This is a battle of wills between your brain and what your brain is telling your body. You can win this battle!

If you have a package of Oreos in the cupboard and a case of Pepsi in the fridge, give it away. You don't need the temptation. While you will need to learn to ignore these choices in the future, the first few days of your detox are not the time to tempt yourself.

It is a good idea to have the entire household detox at the same time. You can support each other as you go through the process of eliminating the sugar in your body and fight your body's demand that you feed it more sugar.

If you need a little encouragement, write yourself little notes and post them on the bathroom mirror, on the pantry door, the refrigerator door or inside your purse where you normally stash your candy bars. One of the benefits of cutting out sugar from your diet is weight loss. If you have been dreaming of being a size smaller, it is a real possibility when you cut out the sugar. Put up a picture of a dress you have been hoping to fit into. Give yourself little reminders about why you are doing the detox.

What to expect as you detox

The first three days of your detox are the toughest. It does get a little easier after that. You can certainly get through 72 hours, right?

Your tastes will change. After the first week of eating no sugar, you will notice food tastes different. You will be able to taste the sweetness in your bread or your favorite herbal tea. Your taste buds will be more aware of the sweetness in a given food or drink.

The first week of your sugar detox can be physically and mentally uncomfortable. However, it is fairly short-lived and the majority of the symptoms subside by the end of the first week. Some people report the following side effects:

- Headache
- Lightheadedness
- Drowsiness
- Grumpiness/crankiness
- Emotional
- Pimples
- Rashes

You are probably looking at that list and thinking, never mind. Sugar cannot be all that bad, right? Wrong. Too much sugar can be very bad. Excessive sugar is actually a serious health issue. All of the above symptoms go away within days or a week. Your body needs time to readjust. Drinking lots of water will help flush your system and eliminate the rashes and pimples that are part of the detox. The headaches will subside within a few days of eliminating sugar as will the lightheadedness. Again, when that headache hits, try drinking a glass of ice water or closing your eyes for a bit.

The emotional side effects like being a little more cranky than usual will also smooth out. One of the main reasons people abuse sugar is because of the emotional response it triggers. It makes you happy to feed your sugar addiction. It is an escape from what may really be troubling you. Depending on the severity of your dependency on sugar as an emotional crutch, you may want to seek out counseling to help you work through the issue that sent you into sugar's arms.

How long will it take to detox and reduce or eliminate cravings?

The cravings will begin to subside within a few days of going cold turkey. Most sugar detox plans are outlined for 21 days. This is because it takes about that long to retrain your body to function without sugar and to train your brain you don't really need it. Some people may get through the rough part of detoxing within a few days, while others will take several weeks to truly get through it. Unfortunately, there is no one size fits all answer to this question. Expect your sugar cravings to subside in no less than three days and no more than 21 days on the high end.

Chapter 4 - What to Eat and What Not to Eat

It can be tricky changing your diet. Sugar in one form or another is added to nearly every ready-to-eat food. Breads, cereals and even fast food all have a little sugar added. You will want to start reading the labels on foods you buy to help you learn more about sugar content.

Good/Bad Carbs

A sugar detox diet may look a little like the Atkins Diet simply because the majority of carbs are eliminated. Unlike the Atkins diet, it isn't all carbs that are considered unhealthy when you are detoxing from sugar. Simple carbohydrates digest quickly and turn into sugar. These are what you want to avoid. The following lists will give you an idea of what are considered good carbs and what are considered bad carbs that should be avoided.

Good Carbs:
- Whole wheat pasta
- Quinoa
- Barley
- Bulgur
- Popcorn
- Fruits and vegetables
- Steel cut oats
- Brown rice

Bad Carbs:
- White bread
- Pasta
- Pizza crust
- Pretzels
- Hamburger/hot dog buns

- Muffins (blueberry, apple bran, banana, etc.)
- Potato chips
- Soda
- Pastries
- Baked goods (cakes, cookies, etc.)

Are supplements recommended?

When you look at the lists of foods you should avoid in order to really detox from sugar, it can be a bit overwhelming. Do not feel bad if the lists are your current daily diet. You are not the only one. But, it is time to make a change. When you start cutting out certain foods you have been eating for years or decades, your body is going to go through a bit of a transition period. You can help lessen the side effects of withdrawal by taking certain supplements.

You don't have to take supplements in order to be healthy, but you can take them to feel better. Many of us rely on sugar to give us that little extra boost first thing in the morning or midday. If your body is healthy and getting all the nutrients it needs, you won't need that sugar boost.

The following are some of the supplements you can take to keep your body on an even keel:

- Fish oil
- Vitamin D
- Multivitamin
- Fiber
- Vitamin B complex [recommended by Dr. Oz to help with withdrawals]
- Chromium picolinate

Your B vitamins are what give you energy. A liquid B12 boost is awesome. Squirt one teaspoon under your tongue in the morning and let it sit there for about 30 seconds. It doesn't taste all that great, but you can feel your body humming once the B12 starts moving through your veins. It will help satisfy that craving for a morning boost of java.

Cinnamon

If you are struggling to manage your blood sugar, especially during and after a sugar detox, a little cinnamon can help do the trick. You don't need to try and gag down a teaspoon of cinnamon every morning. Incorporate it into a few recipes throughout the day and you can safely control your blood sugar without taking any kind of prescription medications. You can even buy it as a supplement at your local grocery store or pharmacy. The effect of cinnamon on blood sugar levels has recently gained the attention of doctors and researchers.

A study[3] proved that regular intake of cinnamon helped lower fasting blood glucose levels by 3 to 5 percent. While that number is not groundbreaking, it is similar to medicines a doctor might prescribe. Imagine being able to control your blood sugar by adding a little cinnamon to your diet? In fact, cinnamon has been used in Chinese medicine for centuries. It isn't a fluke or some crazy snake oil remedy. It truly works.

Identifying "hidden" sugar in your food

There are several different names used for sugar. When you grab a box off the shelf in the supermarket and read the ingredients, you may not find the word sugar in the list. Don't be fooled. There is probably some sugar in there, but it is snuck in under another name. Look for the following ingredients:

- Corn syrup
- Brown sugar

---

[3]http://www.ncbi.nlm.nih.gov/pubmed/?term=Davis+Yokoyama+Cinnamon

- Cane sugar
- Carob syrup
- Dextrose
- Fructose
- Glucose
- Sucrose
- Lactose
- Fruit juice
- Ethyl maltol
- Syrup of any kind is sugar
- Honey
- Molasses

Do not be fooled by a big word that means sugar. It is also important to remember organic sugar is still sugar as well. Just because it is organic doesn't make it any healthier or better for you.

Chapter 5 - Fabulous, *Normal* Sugar Detox Recipes

Alright, this is what you have been waiting for—food recipes. You know the benefits to eliminating refined sugar from your diet along with bad carbohydrates, but what could you possibly eat? These recipes will help you stick to the detox plan.

Don't worry, you will not have to run all over town trying to find some ingredient you have never heard of. These are recipes designed for the average person who doesn't have the time or money to do that. You will need to visit a health food store for some of these ingredients. However, many chain grocery stores are recognizing the need consumers have to eat healthier and most have created a section devoted to organic and natural foods. This is where you will find some of the ingredients, like agave syrup and arrowroot powder, you don't already have in your pantry.

Breakfast

Strawberry Banana Protein Shake
1 banana, frozen
½ cup whole strawberries, frozen
⅔ cup almond milk
½ cup orange juice
1 scoop Formulx Vanilla Protein Powder
½ teaspoon vanilla extract
½ tablespoon ground chia seeds (optional)

Mix all ingredients in a blender and blend until smooth. Perfect for the mornings you are on the go.

Egg and Sausage Cups
2-3 chicken sausage, cooked and chopped
1 red bell pepper, chopped

¼ yellow onion, chopped
8 eggs, whisked
2 garlic cloves, minced
¼ teaspoon garlic powder
⅛ teaspoon red pepper flakes
salt and pepper, to taste

Cook sausage until done in a pan. Mix remaining ingredients in a bowl. Add sausage in. Grease muffin pan or use muffin liners. Pour mixture into each cup and bake at 325 degrees for 35 minutes or until egg is done.

Easy Pancakes
2 bananas, mashed
2 eggs, whisked
½ cup Formulx Vanilla Protein Powder
Enjoy Life Chocolate Chips® (optional – blueberries are also yummy)
1 tablespoon butter or oil

Blend all bananas, eggs and protein powder in a bowl. Add in chocolate chips or other ingredients. Cook on medium heat 2 minutes on each side or until done. Top with fresh fruit or eat plain.

Butternut Squash and Chorizo
1 small butternut squash, peeled and diced small
½ yellow onion, finely diced
½ pound chorizo
salt and pepper, to taste
5 eggs

Cook squash and onion over medium heat until squash is browned on all sides. Add chorizo and cook thoroughly. Add a little salt and pepper to taste. Add eggs into dish. You can scramble the whole thing together or cook eggs over easy inside the hash.

Apple and Orange Slices with Cinnamon

Peel and slice an orange and an apple. Sprinkle with cinnamon. Quick, easy and sweet!

Meaty Quiche

1 pound breakfast pork sausage (or Italian sausage)
1 small sweet potato, diced
½ yellow onion, diced
2 cups fresh spinach
4 eggs, whisked
1 garlic clove, minced
1 teaspoon garlic powder
⅛ teaspoon ground paprika
salt and pepper, to taste
2 tablespoons bacon fat (or other kind of fat)

Press meat into a pie pan to form a crust. Put the meat in the oven and cook at 375 degrees for about 20 minutes. The meat does not have to be cooked all the way through. While meat is cooking, add fat to a saucepan and mix in garlic. Sauté garlic and add in onions and sweet potato. Add a little salt and pepper to the mixture and cook until onions are translucent and potatoes are soft or about 5 minutes. Add in spinach, cover and let cook for about 2 minutes. Remove mixture from heat and pour into a bowl. Let cool before adding eggs, paprika and a dash of salt. Remove meat from oven. Use a paper towel to absorb the grease that has pooled in the crust. Pour egg mixture into meat crust and cook for 23 minutes or until eggs are done. Eggs are done when they are spongy to the touch.

Crockpot Breakfast

8 eggs, whisked
1 sweet potato or yam, shredded
1lb Pork Sausage, broken up
1 yellow onion, diced
1 tablespoon garlic powder
2 teaspoons dried basil

salt and pepper, to taste

Grease bottom of crockpot with coconut oil to keep eggs from sticking. Shred sweet potato and add to crockpot. Add in remaining ingredients and mix well. Place on low setting and cook for 6 to 8 hours.

Lunch

Spicy Turkey Wrap
1 cup extra virgin olive oil
2 medium yellow onions, thinly sliced
8 cloves garlic, minced
2- to 4-inch piece fresh ginger root peeled and minced
4 medium carrots, peeled and shredded
1 tablespoon cayenne pepper
1 tablespoon plus 1 teaspoon ground coriander
1 tablespoon plus 1 teaspoon ground turmeric
1/2 tablespoon ground cinnamon
Salt and freshly ground black pepper, to taste
1 1/4 pounds lean ground turkey
1/2 cup low-sodium chicken broth
1/4 cup finely chopped fresh cilantro

WRAPS

16 large romaine lettuce leaves
2 avocados, peeled, pitted and mashed
2 cups baby spinach
2 cups watercress

Heat oil in a non-stick pan and add onions, garlic and ginger. Sauté for 3 minutes. Add the carrots, cayenne, coriander, turmeric, cinnamon, salt and pepper. Stir together and add in ground turkey. Cook the turkey until is cooked thoroughly, approximately 8 minutes. Pour in chicken broth and mix all ingredients. Remove from heat and add cilantro. Put turkey mixture in a separate bowl.

Place romaine lettuce leaves on a plate. Drop a bit of mashed avocado onto the leaves and spread out. Add spinach and watercress. Top with the spicy turkey mixture. Roll the leaves up and eat!

Egg Salad and Avocado Wraps
1 egg, hard boiled, shell removed
2 egg whites, hard boiled, shell removed
½ ripe avocado
½ teaspoon salt
¼ teaspoon pepper
½ lemon, juice only
¼ cup diced red onion
¼ cup sliced red pepper
¼ cup sliced yellow pepper
4 rice paper wrappers
4 mint leaves

Chop egg up in a bowl. Add in avocado and mash together. Add salt, pepper and lemon juice. Add in red onion and mix well, set aside. Fill a small bowl with warm water. Add one rice paper to the water to soften. Let it sit in water for about a minute. Remove wrapper and place on cutting board. Put a mint leaf inside wrapper and add a few slices of pepper. Add a dollop of avocado mixture to wrapper. Roll up wrapper on each side. Refrigerate until ready to eat.

Creamy Broccoli Soup
2 tablespoons extra virgin olive oil
½ cup diced onion
2 cloves garlic, minced
4 cups broccoli florets
4 cups vegetable broth, low sodium
2 cups fresh spinach
1 avocado
2 tablespoons lemon juice
salt & pepper to taste
optional toppings: fresh parsley, pine nuts, sour cream

Sauté onions and garlic in pan with EVOO. Add broccoli and broth. Bring to a boil, reduce heat and let simmer for 15 minutes. Add spinach to mixture. Remove pit and peel from avocado and mash in a small bowl. Pour lemon juice over avocado. Add avocado to soup mix. Remove from heat and add soup to a blender (immersion if you have it) and blend until smooth.

Shrimp and Avocado Mash
1 pound raw peeled and deveined shrimp
2 tablespoon olive oil (or other fat)
½ tablespoon garlic powder
salt, to taste

Avocado mash

2 avocados, mashed
1 tablespoon hot sauce of choice
juice of 1 lime
juice of ½ a lemon
1 garlic clove, minced
½ small red onion, minced
1/2 cup cilantro, roughly chopped
lots of salt

Line a baking sheet with foil. Add olive oil to a small bowl. Coat shrimp in oil and place on baking sheet. Sprinkle with salt and garlic. Bake at 350 degrees for 15 minutes. While the shrimp is cooking, mix mashed avocadoes, hot sauce, lemon juice, onion and cilantro in a bowl. Serve avocado mash on top of shrimp.

Pork Pitas
1 pound boneless pork loin chops, cut into thin strips
1 tablespoon olive oil
2 teaspoons coarsely ground pepper
2 garlic cloves, minced

1 jar (12 ounces) roasted sweet red peppers, drained and julienned
4 whole wheat pita breads, warmed

Mix pork, olive oil, pepper and garlic in a bowl. Sauté mixture over medium heat in a skillet until pork is cooked. Add in peppers. Mix well. Stuff mixture into pitas. Add sugar-free mayo or caramelized onions for extra flavor.

Turkey Burgers
1/2 cup chopped onion
2 tablespoons reduced-fat plain yogurt
1 tablespoon snipped fresh dill or 1 teaspoon dill weed
1-1/2 teaspoons hot pepper sauce
1/2 teaspoon salt
1 garlic clove, minced
1 pound lean ground turkey
4 whole wheat rolls, split
4 lettuce leaves
4 tomato slices

Combine yogurt, dill, onion, salt, garlic and hot sauce in a bowl. Mix well. Add turkey and mix again. Form patties with the mixture. Cook patties uncovered for 8 minutes on each side or until meat is cooked. Serve on buns with lettuce and tomato.

Quinoa Salad with Tuna
2 tsp extra virgin olive oil
2 tbsp black olives, sliced
1/4 cup tomato, chopped
2 tsp balsamic vinegar
1/4 cup cucumber, chopped
1 cup quinoa
½ cup tuna

Cook the quinoa according to instructions on the package. Allow to cool. Add chopped vegetables to quinoa. Add in tuna (chilled is best) and top with vinegar dressing.

Dinner

Crockpot Chicken Soup
5 lb whole chicken, giblets removed
12 oz of carrots, chopped
4 large scallions, diced
2 tsp sea salt
1 tsp ground ginger
1/2 tsp ground turmeric
1 large bay leaf
2 garlic cloves, minced
6 cups water
1 tbsp apple cider vinegar
2 portabella mushroom caps, chopped

Put carrots, onions and garlic in bottom of crockpot. Add spices and bay leaf. Pour apple cider vinegar in. Place the chicken in the pot with the breast side up. Cook on high for six hours. Turn the chicken over halfway through cooking. Remove the chicken from the pot and remove all of the meat. Put the meat back into the pot and cook for an additional 30 minutes.

Salisbury Steak and Mushroom Gravy
Burgers

2 lbs. Ground beef
1 Egg
2 cloves Garlic
1/2 Yellow onion
1 tsp Garlic powder
1 tsp Onion powder
1 tsp Sea Salt
1 tsp Black pepper

1 tsp Thyme, dried

Gravy
2 tablespoons Fat of your choice (beef, chicken)
3/4 cup Beef broth
1/2 can Coconut milk
1/2 Yellow onion
1 clove Garlic
1 package Mushroom
1 tsp Sea Salt
1 tsp Black pepper
1/2 tsp Garlic powder
1/2 tsp Onion powder

Mix all ingredients for the burgers in a bowl. Use your hands to form patties. Cook the patties on medium heat, about 5 minutes on each side or until done. While the burgers are cooking, make your gravy. In a pan heat the fat, onions and garlic over medium heat. Add in the remaining ingredients and reduce to low heat. Let cook for about 5 minutes or until onions are soft. Pour gravy over the burgers for a delicious dinner.

Meatloaf
1 pound ground beef
10-12 ounces bulk pork breakfast sausage
1 tablespoon bacon fat (or other fat)
2 garlic cloves, minced
1 yellow onion, diced
1 medium zucchini, diced
4 ounces of button mushrooms, sliced
2 tablespoons dried parsley
2 tablespoons dried basil
1 teaspoon garlic powder
salt and pepper, to taste

Put fat in frying pan and add onions and garlic. When onions are almost translucent, add in zucchini. Cook for 3 minutes before adding in mushrooms. Cook for an additional 4 minutes. Once veggies are soft, add in spices and seasonings. Remove from heat and allow to cool. Place veggie mixture in a bowl and add in ground beef and sausage. Use your hands to blend everything together.

Line a bread pan with foil. It helps to spray the foil with a cooking spray. Put the meat mixture in the pan and spread it out evenly. Bake at 400 degrees for about 40 minutes or until meat is done.

Chicken Enchilada Bake
coconut oil, for greasing baking dish
1 pound cooked, shredded chicken
1 (14 ounce) can enchilada sauce
1 (6 ounce) can of diced green chiles
1 orange bell pepper, seeded and diced
¼ red onion, diced
2 garlic cloves, minced
¼ teaspoon chili powder
¼ teaspoon dried oregano
salt and pepper, to taste
3 eggs, whisked
cilantro, to garnish

Mix all ingredients except for eggs and cilantro in a large bowl. Stir in eggs. Pour into 8x8 baking dish greased with coconut oil. Cook for 1 hour at 350 degrees. Check to see if eggs are thoroughly cooked. If not, cook for an additional 15 minutes. Top with cilantro.

Chicken and Bacon Bowls
4 pieces of bacon, diced
2 garlic cloves, minced
½ yellow onion, minced
1.5 pounds chicken, cut into 1 inch cubes
1 (14 ounce) can of diced tomatoes, drained
2 (6 ounce) cans of diced green chiles

1 small head of cauliflower, riced
½ teaspoon chili powder
½ teaspoon red pepper flakes
salt and pepper, to taste

Add bacon to a large pot and cook until crispy. Remove bacon and put on paper towel. Leave 3 to 4 tablespoons of fat in pot and toss the rest. Add garlic, chicken and onion to the pot and cook over medium heat until chicken is cooked. Add tomatoes, chilies and cauliflower. Add salt and mix well. Add chili powder and red pepper and mix well. Let simmer over medium heat for 10 minutes. Add in bacon pieces. Serve immediately. Top with avocado and green onions.

Creamy Dill Salmon Fillets
2 salmon filets (6 ounces each)
¼ cup Sir Kensington's Mayo or 30 Second Mayo
1 tablespoon minced fresh dill
¼ teaspoon garlic powder
salt and pepper, to taste

Line baking sheet with parchment paper. Place fillets on sheet and sprinkle with salt. Mix mayo, dill, garlic, salt and pepper in a small bowl. Coat the tops of the fillets with the mayo mixture. Cook at 450 degrees for about 8 minutes.

Beef Stir Fry
1 cup coconut aminos (or gluten free soy sauce)
½ cup orange juice
3 tablespoons honey
1 teaspoon fish sauce
2 garlic cloves, minced
1 teaspoons fresh ginger, grated
½ teaspoon red pepper flakes
3 tablespoons arrowroot powder
1 pound flank steak, thinly sliced against the grain
3 crowns of broccoli, cut into florets
salt and pepper, to taste

2 tablespoons of coconut oil
½ cup toasted cashews

In a small bowl, mix together the coconut or soy sauce, OJ, honey, fish sauce, garlic, ginger, red pepper and arrowroot powder. In another bowl, place the sliced beef and pour the mixture over the top. Put the beef in the fridge for 30 minutes.

Place a pan on medium heat and add a tablespoon of coconut oil. Add broccoli and salt. Add a teaspoon of water and cover to allow broccoli to get soft. Once broccoli is cooked to desired softness, remove from pan and set aside. Add another tablespoon of coconut oil to the pan and heat on medium. Add in the beef strips. Cook until beef is almost cooked through. Add broccoli back to the pan and add in cashews. Cook another minute and serve hot.

Chapter 6 - Strategies to Stay On Track For Good

Once you have successfully completed a sugar detox, you will start to feel better as well as look better. Although a detox is only a short-term thing, you can choose to stay away from sugar forever. It is too easy to get sucked back into sugary ways, especially around the holidays and other special occasions. You can stay sugar free and remain healthy and feeling good by following some of these tips and tricks:

*When you do decide to do a sugar detox, try and avoid planning it around the holidays. If you know you are going to be attending several Christmas or New Year's Eve parties, cut back on sugar, but wait to do the detox until after the parties are over. You don't want to tempt yourself that much. If you fail, you are going to assume it is too difficult and you may not try again. It **CAN** be done.

*Make meals and snacks ahead. If you are off on Sunday, make up a pot of one of the soups from above. Store it in the refrigerator so you have a quick dinner or lunch and are not tempted to grab a sugary snack to appease your hunger. You can do this with treats as well.

*Eat a diet that is rich in protein. This will help curb sugar cravings. When your body has everything it needs to be healthy, it won't send out signals for foods that are unhealthy, like refined sugars and carbohydrates.

*When you get a strong sugar craving, try eating something sour. Sauerkraut is an excellent choice. It combats that sugar craving and is good for the flora in your gut.

*Keep dried fruit or fresh fruit, if possible, at work or on hand. This is a quick way to satisfy a sugar craving.

*Drink ice water with a slice of lemon or sprig of mint when you get a craving for an ice cold soda. Staying hydrated can help eliminate the need for a cold, sugary drink.

*Season your foods with cinnamon to help satisfy that sugar craving without actually consuming sugar.

*Clean out the pantry, refrigerator and freezer. Remove sugary food that will scream at you to try just one bite.

*Make sure you get plenty of sleep every night. When you are exhausted, your body is depleted of its energy stores and will demand sugar to fuel it up.

*Reward yourself when you make it 2 weeks, 4 weeks or whatever length of time you decide. Give yourself a makeover, buy new clothes or spend a day at the beach. Whatever reward will motivate you.

*Pack your lunch instead of trying to navigate a restaurant menu. This gives you full control over your meal and you won't be limited to a plain Caesar salad for lunch.

Conclusion

Well, you've reached the end of the book. Have you started to detox yet? If not, do it now! There's no time like the present and the sooner you start the sooner you will be on the road to better health with increased energy. If you have started I wish you much success as you move forward in the process. It does get easier so take it seriously and make it happen!

As I mentioned in the introduction, once you complete your detox, go back to chapter 1 and re-take the short quiz to see where you stand with sugar in your diet. Compare the answers with the first time you took it and I know you will be surprised at the outcome.

Finally, if you enjoyed this book, please take the time to share your thoughts and post a review on Amazon. I would greatly appreciate it!

Thank you and good luck!

PS: You may also be interested in my other books. Get them on Amazon today!

Atkins Diet Essentials: Turbocharge Your Weight Loss with this New and Improved Version of Atkins' Classic Diet Plan

DASH Diet Essentials: A Beginner's Guide to the DASH Diet with a Proven Lifestyle Plan and Delicious Recipes so You can Lower Your Blood Pressure, Lose Weight, Feel Great and Live a Healthy Life

These are all great resources I created to help you on your way to better health. It's part of my Healthy Life Series.

References

http://www.webmd.com/diet/ss/slideshow-sugar-addiction

http://www.merriam-webster.com/dictionary/addiction

http://www.huffingtonpost.com/2013/10/29/sugar-addiction-drug_n_4173632.html

http://www.fitwatch.com/weight-loss/signs-that-you-may-be-addicted-to-sugar-749.html

http://drhyman.com/blog/2013/06/27/5-clues-you-are-addicted-to-sugar/#close

https://shine.yahoo.com/team-mom/5-surprising-signs-youre-sugar-addict-204200194.html

http://www.sheerbalance.com/brettsblog/3-reasons-you-crave-sugar-that-have-nothing-to-do-with-food/

http://www.thehealthsite.com/fitness/why-do-we-crave-sweets/

http://www.huffingtonpost.com/2013/06/29/fruit-sugar-versus-white-sugar_n_3497795.html

http://www.mayoclinic.org/healthy-living/nutrition-and-healthy-eating/in-depth/artificial-sweeteners/art-20046936

http://www.webmd.com/food-recipes/features/are-artificial-sweeteners-safe

http://www.ehow.com/about_5300807_sugar-detox-side-effects.html

http://endsugaraddiction.com/expert-tips/

http://drhyman.com/blog/2014/03/06/top-10-big-ideas-detox-sugar/

http://www.fitsugar.com/Other-Names-Sugar-Appear-Labels-810571

http://healthyeating.sfgate.com/list-good-carbs-bad-carbs-6520.html

http://abcnews.go.com/GMA/dr-mehmet-oz-beat-fat-sugar-addiction-detox/story?id=12823912

http://www.nydailynews.com/life-style/health/day-4-news-sugar-detox-series-article-1.1610361

http://www.feedtheclan.com/family-chow-102913-also-cold-fighting-chicken-soup-recipe/

http://paleomg.com/category/breakfast/

http://www.recipe4living.com/articles/top_10_sugar_free_dessert_recipes.htm

http://www.sugarfreemom.com/

http://www.tasteofhome.com/recipes/healthy-eating/diabetic-recipes/diabetic-sandwich-recipes

http://www.fatsecret.com/recipes/collections/nutrition/sugar-free/Lunch.aspx

http://www.sugarfreemom.com/recipes/25-back-to-school-healthy-kid-friendly-snacks/

http://www.mnn.com/food/healthy-eating/blogs/12-tips-for-kicking-the-refined-sugar-habit

www.ingramcontent.com/pod-product-compliance
Lightning Source LLC
Chambersburg PA
CBHW070243290526
45789CB00004B/1744